Keto Diet Easy Cookbook

Easy And Delicious Keto Cookbook For Effortless Weight Loss

Elena Harrison

Table of Contents

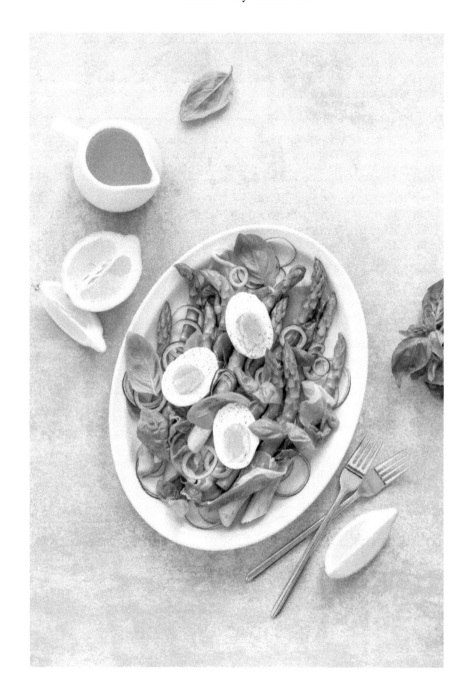

INTRODUCTION

The ketogenic diet has been highly praised and praised for the benefits of weight loss. This high-fat, low-carb diet has been shown to be extremely healthy overall. It really makes your body burn fat, like a talking machine. Public figures appreciate it too. But the question is, how does ketosis enhance weight loss? The following is a detailed picture of the ketosis and weight loss process.

Some people consider ketosis to be abnormal. Although it has been approved by many nutritionists and doctors. many people still disapprove of it. The misconceptions are due to the myths that have spread around the ketogenic diet.

Once your body is out of glucose, it automatically depends on stored fat. It is also important to understand that carbohydrates produce glucose and once you start a low carbohydrate diet, you will also be able to lower your glucose levels. Then your body will produce fuel through fat, instead of carbohydrates, that is, glucose.

The process of accumulating fat through fat is known as ketosis, and once your body enters this state, it becomes extremely effective at burning unwanted fat. Also, since glucose levels are low during the ketogenic diet, your body achieves many other health benefits.

A ketogenic diet is not only beneficial for weight loss, but it also helps improve your overall health in a positive way. Unlike all other diet plans, which focus on reducing calorie intake, ketogenic focuses on putting your body in a natural metabolic state, that is, ketosis. The only factor that makes this diet questionable is that this nature of metabolism is not very well thought out. By getting tattoos on your body regularly, your body will quickly burn stored fat, leading to great weight loss.

Now the question arises. How does ketosis affect the human body?

However, this phase does not last more than 2-3 days. This is the time it takes for the human body to enter the ketosis phase. Once you get in, you won't have any side effects.

You should also start gradually reducing your calorie and carbohydrate intake. The most common mistake dietitians make is that they tend to start eliminating everything from their diet at the same time. This is where the problem arises. The human body will react extremely negatively when you limit everything at once. You must start gradually. Read this guide to learn more about how to approach the ketogenic diet after 50.

Most fats are good and essential for our health so there are essential fatty acids and essential amino acids (proteins). Fat is the most efficient form of energy, and each gram contains about 9 calories. This more than doubles the amount of carbohydrates and protein (both have 4 calories per gram).

When you eat a lot of fat and protein and significantly reduce carbohydrates, your body adjusts and converts the fat and protein, as well as the fat that it has stored, into ketones or ketones, for energy. This metabolic process is called ketosis. This is where the ketogen in the ketogenic diet comes from.

BREAKFAST

1. Zucchini Spread

Preparation time: 5 minutes

Cooking time: 15 minutes

Servings: 4

Ingredients:

- 4 zucchinis, roughly chopped
- 1 tablespoon sweet paprika
- Salt and black pepper to the taste
- 1 tablespoon butter, melted

DIRECTIONS:

1. Grease a baking pan that fits the Air Fryer with the butter, add all the ingredients, toss, and cook at 360 degrees F for 15 minutes.
2. Transfer to a blender, pulse well, divide into bowls and serve for breakfast.

Nutrition: Calories 240 Fat 14 Fiber 2 carbohydrates 5 Protein 11

2. Garlic Cheese Bread Loaf

Preparation time: 10 minutes

Cooking time: 45 minutes

Servings: 10

Ingredients:

- 1 tbsp parsley, chopped
- ½ cup butter, unsalted and softened
- 2 tbsp garlic powder
- 6 large eggs
- ½ tsp oregano seasoning
- 1 tsp baking powder
- 2 cups almond flour
- ½ tsp xanthan gum
- 1 cup cheddar cheese, shredded
- ½ tsp salt

Directions:

- Preheat the oven to 355F.
- Line a baking pan with parchment paper.
- In a food blender, pulse the eggs until smooth. Then combine the butter and pulse for 1 minute more.
- Blend the almond flour and baking powder for 90 seconds or until thickens.
- Finally, combine the garlic, oregano, parsley, and cheese until mixed.

- Pour into the prepared and bake in the oven for 45 minutes.

- Cool, slice, and serve.

Nutrition: Calories: 299 Fat: 27g Carb: 4g Protein: 11g

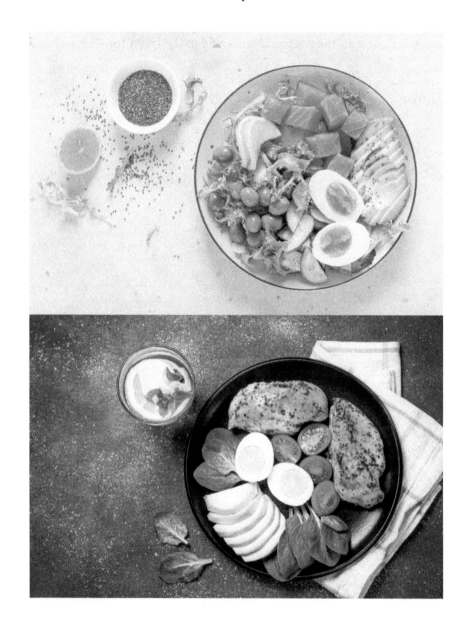

KETO BREAD

3. Keto Kalamata Olive Loaf

Preparation Time: 2 hours

Cooking Time: 10 minutes

Total Time: 2 hours 10 minutes

Servings: 10 slices

Ingredients

- ½ cup brine from olives
- cup warm water
- tbsps. olive oil
- 1 ½ tsp. salt
- tbsps. sugar
- cups almond flour
- 1 2/3 cup almond meal
- 1 ½ tsp. dried basil leaves
- 2 tsps. active dry yeast
- ½ cup olives finely chopped

Directions

1. Combine the brine and warm water.
2. Using the bread bucket, put all ingredients except olives in the order of their appearance on the ingredient list starting with the brine mixture.

3. Select the WHEAT BREAD cycle on your machine. If there is no WHEAT BREAD cycle, you can select BASIC cycle. Close the cover and press START.

4. With the first beep of the machine, open the lid and add in the olives. Close the lid and let the cycle continue.

5. When the cycle ends, you can take the loaf out and let it cool in a cooling rack.

6. Slice before serving.

Nutrition: Calories: 161 Calories from fat: 130 Total Fat: 14 g Total Carbohydrates: 8 g Net Carbohydrates: 5 g Protein: 5 g

4. <u>Coconut Cloud Bread</u>

Preparation time: 10 minutes

Cooking time: 25 minutes

Servings: 4

Ingredients:

- 3 eggs

- 3 tbsp. coconut cream

- 1/2 tsp. baking powder

- Optional toppings:

- sea salt

- black pepper

- rosemary

Direction:

1. First, separate the egg yolks and egg whites.

2. Beat egg yolks in a bowl.

3. Stir in cream and continue beating with a hand mixer until creamy and smooth.

4. Beat the egg whites with baking powder in another bowl until it forms peaks.

5. Quickly add yolk mixture to the whites and mix well until fluffy.

6. Spread ¼ of the batter on to a baking sheet separately to make 4 circles.

7. Bake the batter for 25 minutes approximately at 350 degrees F.

8. Serve.

Nutrition: Calories 158 Total Fat 15.2 g Saturated Fat 5.2 g Cholesterol 269 mg Sodium 178 mg Total Carbs 3.4 g Sugar 1.1 g Fiber 3.5 g Protein 5.5 g

5. <u>Rosemary and Garlic Bread</u>

Preparation time: 10 minutes

Cooking time: 50 minutes

Servings: 8

Ingredients:

- 1/2 cup coconut flour

- stick butter (8 tbsp.)

- 6 large eggs

- 1 tsp. baking powder

- tsp. dried rosemary

- 1/2-1 tsp. garlic powder

- 1/2 tsp. onion powder

- 1/4 tsp. pink Himalayan salt

Direction:

1. Start by whisking rosemary, salt, garlic, onion, baking powder, and coconut flour in a bowl.

2. Beat eggs in a mixing bowl until creamy.

3. Now, put butter in a large bowl and melt it in the microwave.

4. Slowly stir in the whisked eggs and continue beating with a hand mixer.

5. Now, whisk in the dry mixture and mix well until well incorporated.

6. Spread the batter in an 8x4 inch loaf pan and bake it for 50 minutes approximately at 350 degrees F.

7. Slice and serve with butter on top.

Nutrition: Calories 214 Total Fat 19 g Saturated Fat 5.8 g Cholesterol 15 mg Sodium 123 mg Total Carbs 3.5 g Sugar 1.9 g Fiber 2.1 g Protein 6.5 g

6. Psyllium Husk Bread

Preparation time: 10 minutes

Cooking time: 35 minutes

Servings: 10

Ingredients:

- 1/2 cup coconut flour
- 2 tbsp. psyllium husk powder
- 1/2 tsp. baking powder
- 1/4 tsp. pink Himalayan salt
- 3/4 cup water
- 4 large eggs
- 4 tbsp. butter

Direction:

1. Start by whisking the husk powder, salt, baking powder, and coconut flour in a bowl.
2. Beat eggs with water and melted butter in a mixer until it's smooth.
3. Slowly stir in the dry mixture and mix well until smooth.
4. Make 10 dinner rolls out of this bread dough and place the dough on a baking sheet.

5. Bake them for 35 minutes, approximately, at 350 degrees F until all done.

6. Slice and serve.

Nutrition: Calories 220 Total Fat 20.1 g Saturated Fat 7.4 g Cholesterol 132 mg Sodium 157 mg

Total Carbs 3.3 g Sugar 0.4 g Fiber 2.4 g Protein 6.1 g

7. <u>Parsley Cheddar Bread</u>

Preparation time: 10 minutes

Cooking time: 4 minutes

Servings: 2

Ingredients:

- tbsp. butter
- tbsp. coconut flour
- 1 large egg
- 1 tbsp. heavy whipping cream
- tbsp. water
- 1/4 cup cheddar cheese
- 1/8 tsp. garlic powder
- 1/8 tsp. onion powder
- 1/8 tsp. dried parsley
- 1/8 tsp. pink Himalayan salt
- 1/8 tsp. black pepper
- 1/4 tsp. baking powder

Direction:

1. Melt the butter by heating it in a coffee mug for 20 seconds.
2. Slowly stir in seasonings, baking powder, and coconut flour. Mix well using a fork until smooth.
3. Whisk in cream, cheese, water, and egg.
4. Beat well until smooth then bake for 3 minutes in the microwave.

5. Allow the bread to cool then serve.

Nutrition: Calories 113 Total Fat 8.4 g Saturated Fat 12.1 g Cholesterol 27 mg Sodium 39 mg Total Carbs 4.2 g Sugar 3.1 g Fiber 4.6 g Protein 8.1 g

8. Garlic Focaccia Bread

Preparation time: 10 minutes

Cooking time: 20 minutes

Servings: 4

Ingredients:

- Dry Ingredients
- cup almond flour
- ¼ cup coconut flour
- ½ tsp. xanthan gum
- 1 tsp. garlic powder
- 1 tsp. flaky salt
- ½ tsp. baking soda
- ½ tsp. baking powder
- Wet Ingredients
- eggs
- 1 tbsp. lemon juice
- tsp. olive oil + 2 tbsp. olive oil to drizzle

Direction:

1. Start by preheating the oven to 350 degrees F.
2. Layer a baking sheet with parchment paper.
3. Now, whisk all the dry ingredients in a bowl.
4. Beat lemon juice, oil, and egg in a bowl until well incorporated.
5. Whisk in dry ingredients and mix well until it forms a dough.

6. Spread the dough on a baking sheet and cover it with aluminum foil.

7. Bake for 10 minutes approximately then remove the foil.

8. Drizzle olive oil on top and bake for another 10 minutes uncovered.

9. Garnish with basil and Italian seasoning.

10. Serve.

Nutrition: Calories 301 Total Fat 26.3 g Saturated Fat 14.8 Cholesterol 322 mg Sodium 597 mg Total Carbs 2.6 g Fiber 0.6 g Sugar 1.9 g Protein 12 g

9. <u>Keto Yeast Loaf Bread</u>

Preparation Time: 5 minutes

Cooking Time: 4 hours

Total Time: 4 hours 5 minutes

Servings: 16 slices (1 slice per serving)

Ingredients

- package dry yeast
- ½ tsp. sugar
- 1 1/8 cup warm water about 90-100 degrees F
- tbsps. Olive oil or avocado oil
- 1 cup vital wheat gluten flour
- ¼ cup oat flour
- ¾ cup soy flour
- ¼ cup flax meal
- ¼ cup wheat bran course, unprocessed
- 1 tbsp. sugar
- 1 ½ tsp. baking powder
- 1 tsp. salt

Directions

1. Mix the sugar, water and yeast in the bread bucket to proof the yeast. If the yeast does not bubble, toss and replace it.

2. Combine all the dry ingredients in a bowl and mix thoroughly. Pour over the wet ingredients in the bread bucket.

3. Set the bread machine and select BASIC cycle to bake the loaf. Close the lid. This takes 3 to 4 hours.

4. When the cycle ends, remove the bread from the bread machine.

5. Cool on a rack before slicing.

6. Serve with butter or light jam.

Nutrition: Calories: 99 Calories from fat: 45 Total Fat: 5 g Total Carbohydrates: 7 g Net Carbohydrates: 5 g Protein: 9 g

10.Macadamia Nut Bread

Preparation time: 10 minutes

Cooking time: 40 minutes

Servings: 6

Ingredients:

- 5 oz. macadamia nuts
- 5 large eggs
- ¼ cup coconut flour
- ½ tsp. baking soda
- ½ tsp. apple cider vinegar

Direction:

1. Start by preheating the oven to 350 degrees F.
2. Blend macadamia nuts in a food processor until it forms a nut butter.
3. Continue blending while adding eggs one by one until well incorporated.
4. Stir in apple cider vinegar, baking soda, and coconut flour.
5. Blend until well mixed and incorporated.
6. Grease a bread pan with cooking spray and spread the batter in a pan.

7. Bake the batter for 40 minutes approximately until golden brown.

8. Slice and serve.

Nutrition: Calories 248 Total Fat 19.3 g Saturated Fat 4.8 g Cholesterol 32 mg Sodium 597 mg Total Carbs 3.1 g Fiber 0.6 g Sugar 1.9 g Protein 7.9 g

11. Buttery Flatbread

Preparation time: 10 minutes

Cooking time: 8 minutes

Servings: 4

Ingredients:

- cup almond flour
- tbsp. coconut flour
- tsp. xanthan gum
- 1/2 tsp. baking powder
- 1/2 tsp. flaky salt
- 1 whole egg + 1 egg white
- 1 tbsp. water
- 1 tbsp. oil, for frying
- 1 tbsp. melted butter, for slathering

Direction:

1. Start by whisking baking powder, salt, flours, and xanthan gum in a bowl.
2. Beat egg whites and egg in a bowl until creamy.
3. Fold in flour mixture and mix until well incorporated.
4. Add a tablespoon of water to the dough and cut it into 4 equal parts.
5. Spread each part out into a flatbread and cook each for 1 minute per side in a skillet with oil.

6. Garnish with butter, parsley, and salt.

7. Serve.

Nutrition: Calories 216 Total Fat 20.9 g Saturated Fat 8.1 g Cholesterol 241 mg Total Carbs 4.3 g Sugar 1.8 g Fiber 3.8 g Sodium 8 mg Protein 6.4 g

12. Everyday White Bread

Preparation time: 10 minutes or less

Cooking time: 20 minutes

Ingredients

- 8 slices / 1 pound
- ¾ cup water, at 80°F to 90°F
- tablespoon melted butter, cooled
- 1 tablespoon sugar
- ¾ teaspoon salt
- tablespoons skim milk powder
- cups white bread flour
- ¾ teaspoon bread machine or instant yeast
- 12 slices / 1½ pounds
- 1⅛ cups water, at 80°F to 90°F
- 1½ tablespoons melted butter, cooled
- 1½ tablespoons sugar
- 1 teaspoon salt
- tablespoons skim milk powder
- 3 cups white bread flour
- 1¼ teaspoons bread machine or instant yeast
- 16 slices / 2 pounds
- 1½ cups water, at 80°F to 90°F
- 2 tablespoons melted butter, cooled
- 2 tablespoons sugar

- 2 teaspoons salt
- ¼ cup skim milk powder
- cups white bread flour
- 1½ teaspoons bread machine or instant yeast

Directions

1. Place the ingredients in your bread machine as recommended by the manufacturer.
2. Program the machine for Basic/White bread, select light or medium crust, and press Start.
3. When the loaf is done, remove the bucket from the machine.
4. Let the loaf cool for 5 minutes.
5. Gently shake the bucket to remove the loaf, and turn it out onto a rack to cool.
6. "Did You Know?" Powdered milk is usually made from skim milk. This is because the fat particles in regular milk could go rancid, shortening the shelf life of powdered milk, despite the fact that all the water has been removed. Whenever possible, smell the powdered milk, and if there is any odor at all, do not buy it.

Nutrition: Calories: 140 Total fat: 2g Saturated fat: 1g Carbohydrates: 27g Fiber: 1g Sodium: 215mg Protein: 4g

KETO PASTA

13.Garganelli all'Uovo Fatti in Casa (Homemade Egg Garganelli)

Preparation time: 10 minutes

Cooking time: 60 minutes

Serves: 8

Ingredients:

- 100 g durum wheat semolina
- 250 g 00 flour
- Water
- Re-milled semolina for dusting
- 3 eggs
- 2 tbsp. extra virgin olive oil
- Salt to taste

Directions:

1. Homemade egg Garganelli first way:
2. Make the dough for the garganelli by hand: sift the flours and pour them on a pastry board. Make a hole in the center, where you will break the eggs, add the salt and extra virgin olive oil.
3. Start by beating the eggs with a fork, and slowly taking some flour. Then continue to knead with your hands, add a little water (just enough) to obtain a workable dough, but not too soft. Knead until it is smooth and elastic. It will take about 10

minutes. Wrap the dough with plastic wrap and let it rest for at least 1/2 hour.

4. After resting, cut the dough in half. The part you don't use right away, keep it wrapped in cling film, and then roll it out later.

5. Roll out the dough with a rolling pin, until you get a thin sheet.

6. With a wheel cut the dough so as to obtain many squares of about 4 cm each side. Cover them with cling film to keep them from drying out.

7. Take one square of pasta at a time, and with the help of the wooden stick, roll it up on itself, starting from the corner. Turn it by pressing lightly on the pastry board, so that the pasta closes well. Pass it on the rigagnocchi. If you have the special tool for garganelli you can train it directly above.

8. Remove the garganelli from the stick and place it on a dripping pan lined with parchment paper. Proceed in the same way to make all the garganelli.

9. You can cook them immediately, or you can keep them for a few days, simply covered with a clean cloth.

Nutrition: Calories: 387 Sugar: 3 g Fat: 12 g Carbohydrates: 1 g Fiber: 3 g Protein: 59 g.

14. Busiate Trapanesi (Busiate from Trapani)

Preparation time: 1 hour

Cooking time: 5 minutes

Serves: 10

Ingredients

- 400 ml water
- 2 tbsp. extra virgin olive oil
- 1 kg Durum wheat semolina
- 2 tsp. salt

Directions:

1. On the wooden pastry board, pour the semolina, in the center, make a bowl and put some little water, oil and salt.

2. Begin kneading by slowly adding the water that is needed. Knead until an elastic and smooth mixture has been obtained. Leave to rest for 1 hour.

3. When you use the planetary mixer, put all ingredients apart from water that is required to be poured slowly. Working on the dough by the planetary mixer takes about 10 minutes for one to get a great result of pasta.

4. It's now time to make the busiate. Make small rolls from the cut small pasta pieces like thin breadsticks and cut them 10 cm long. Diagonally putting the wooden skewer over the roll end,

twist the dough around it and form a curl. By sliding out, remove the busiate and keep using all the pasta.

Nutrition: Calories: 390 Sugar: 5 g Fat: 11 g Carbohydrates: 2 g Fiber: 3 g Protein: 45 g.

15. Maltagliati

Preparation time: 1 hour

Cooking time: 2 minutes

Serves: 4

Ingredients

- All-purpose flour
- Sea salt
- Water

Directions:

1. To make the pasta

2. Use the All-purpose flour to dust the baking sheets.

3. Mix the flour and salt and add water. Use your hands to combine to form dough. Pass the dough through the pasta machine on the widest setting. Use a knife to cut if it becomes very long.

4. Alternatively, you can use a rolling pin to press and make the dough thin.

5. Using a knife cut out your dough into 6-by-4-inch sheets.

6. Dust the pasta sheets with flour and let them rest for 5 minutes so they are not too sticky.

7. Put them one on top of the other (maximum three sheets) and, using a sharp knife, cut the pasta sheets into 11/2- to 2-inch irregular shapes resembling a rhombus.

8. Separate the cut pasta and transfer to the baking sheets.

9. Repeat the process until all dough is finished.

10. Cooking the pasta

11. Bring salted water to boil in a large saucepan. Cook the pasta until al dente, or for 3 minutes. Take a bite to test this.

12. After 3 minutes, use a slotted spoon to remove the pasta and remove the excess water by shaking gently.

13. Serve immediately with the sauce of your choice.

14. You can use tools and equipment like, Pasta machine or rolling pin, Knife, no serrated, 3 baking sheets, Large pot, Wooden spoon, Slotted spoon

Nutrition: Calories: 387 Sugar: 3 g Fat: 12 g Carbohydrates: 2 g Fiber: 3 g Protein: 45 g.

16.Ravioli del Plin

Preparation time: 2 hours

Cooking time: 1 hour 30 minutes

Serves: 8

Ingredients:

- 4 eggs
- 400 g flour
- For the stuffing:
- 1 large onion
- 1 egg
- 30 g spinach
- 200 g pork loin
- 200 g rabbit legs
- 300 g carrots
- 250 g calf pulp
- 100 g celery
- 30 g escarole
- Vegetable broth
- Extra virgin olive oil
- 15 g parmesan cheese
- Salt
- Pepper to taste

Directions:

1. Put the flour on the work surface and break the eggs inside, one at a time. Mix the eggs using a spoon, starting form the

inside. Knead the dough using a fork or with your hands and mix all the flour. If the dough is a bit hard, add few tablespoons of water and continue kneading until its compact and smooth.

2. Using a cling film, cover the pasta and leave it to rest in a cool and dry place for an hour.

3. Cut celery, onions and carrots and set them aside. Remove the veal pulp and the fat part of the loin. You can as well ask the butcher to clean the meat for you by removing the parts that have fats.

4. Heat a few tablespoons of oil in a large saucepan and fry the veal pulp and pork loin until golden brown. Add 2 tablespoons of oil in another pan and fry the rabbit eggs till they are brown.

5. When they are well browned, add the meat, celery, carrots, onions, pepper and salt in a single pan and add water or a ladle of broth. Cover them and cook for 1 hour. If it's necessary, add water or broth during the cooking process.

6. When the meat is ready, remove and let it cool. Keep the cooking juices with the vegetables aside for use in dressing the ravioli. Meanwhile, in a separate pan, add some oil and cook the escarole and spinach until they are wilted. This takes about 5 minutes. If you want, you can cook the endive and spinach in a single pan but first cook the endive for few minutes and add the spinach later since it takes less time.

7. In the meantime, cut the veal meat, pork loin and bone the rabbit into pieces and put all the meats in a mixer. Cut them and add the vegetables, cheese and the egg. Season it with pepper and salt and if it is necessary, add a little broth.

8. Blend all the ingredients together till you get a very compact and dense filling.

9. Now start preparing the ravioli del plin. Take some dough and roll out the thin sheet. On half of the bottom sheet, put half a ball of filling about 20 g and between them, leave a space of 1-2 cm. Quickly work on the dough to avoid it from hardening.

10. Fold the pasta on itself and pinch the edges of the dough on the sides with the fingers, from the long side. Cut the pasta lengthwise few millimeters from the filling using a wheel cut and then separate the ravioli and give it a rectangular shape.

11. Get a tray with a cloth dusted with flour and put the ravioli. Take the previously stewed vegetables and place them in a mixer and blend them till you get a homogeneous and smooth sauce.

12. In abundant salted water, cook the ravioli del plin for few minutes. Drain and season with the sauce obtained from the cooking surface of the meat as soon as they rise to the surface.

13. Serve and enjoy your ravioli del plin.

Nutrition: Calories: 387 Sugar: 3 g Fat: 12 g Carbohydrates: 2 g Fiber: 3 g Protein: 45 g.

17.Cappelletti

Preparation time: 60 minutes

Cooking time: 20 minutes

Serves: 6

Ingredients:

- For egg pasta:
- 4 eggs
- 400 g 00 flour
- For the stuffing:
- 50 g celery
- 60 g carrots
- 150 g pork, minced
- 50 g parmesan, grated
- 50 g red wine
- 30 g extra virgin olive oil
- 100 g chicken breast
- 100 g veal, minced
- 1 egg
- 60 g golden onions
- Nutmeg
- Black pepper
- Salt

Directions:

1. Start by preparing the egg pasta. In a large bowl, pour the flour, add the lightly beaten eggs and flour.

2. Use your hands to knead until you get homogeneous and smooth dough, which you will leave to rest at room temperature after wrapping it in a plastic bag for 30 minutes.

3. Meanwhile, be preparing the filling. Cut the carrots, celery and onions and pour in a large pan with oil. Let it stew for like 10 minutes while often stirring.

4. Cut the chicken into tubes and use a knife to chop finely and then add the initial stir-fry with the minced pork and veal.

5. Use a wooden spoon to stir for 6 minutes and then blend with red wine.

6. Once the alcohol evaporates, add the pepper and salt and cook for 4-5 minutes. Pour the meat that is cooked in the mixer and get a mixture that is finer.

7. Transfer the lightly beaten egg and the grated parmesan into a container. Add ground black pepper, salt and nutmeg and then mix. Keep aside.

8. Remove the film and roll out with a rolling pin or a pasta machine after taking the egg pasta. Roll on a lightly floured pastry board. Slightly flatten the dough, flour it lightly and put it between two rollers if you are using a pasta machine.

9. It is crucial to always begin from the widest thickness till you get to the narrow one adding a pinch of flour on each side each time. During this operation, sometimes the dough

deforms and you have to fold it by pulling one flap then the other towards the center.

10. Finally, slightly squeeze in the middle and begin pulling the dough between the rollers again. Get thin sheets of about 0.6 mm and cover them with plastic wraps to avoid drying out as a result of much air

11. Then cut 5 cm squares of dough with a 24 smooth wheel that you will fill with a teaspoon of compound. Try to position the seasoning well by compacting it in the center and fold the opposite end and form a triangle. Pull the two ends towards you and join them.

12. Flatten down and join them slightly pinching with your fingers. Since they tend to open while you are cooking, make sure they are closed tightly. Repeat this operation for all the others until you get all the cappelletti ready to be cooked.

13. While you prepare them, lay them on a tray where you will have put a lightly floured dish and clean cloth with semolina.

Nutrition: Calories: 387 Sugar: 3 g Fat: 12 g Carbohydrates: 2 g Fiber: 3 g Protein: 45 g.

18. Caramelle Ricotta e Spinaci (Ricotta and Spinach Candies)

Preparation time: 90 minutes

Cooking time: 20 minutes

Serves: 4

Ingredients:

- For egg pasta:
- 2 eggs
- 250 g 00 flour
- 1 yolk
- For the stuffing:
- 1 pinch, nutmeg
- 250 g spinach
- 50 g parmesan
- 125 g cow's milk ricotta
- Black pepper
- Salt
- For the dressing
- Parmesan cheese
- 6 leaves, sage
- 100 g butter

Directions:

1. Preparing the ricotta and spinach candies, you start with egg pasta. In a bowl, pour the flour and keep about 50 g to add if

need be, add eggs and do everything inside one bowl. Once the eggs are absorbed, continue handling the dough on a work surface until its elastic and smooth.

2. Give it a spherical shape once they are ready and let them rest in a cook place with lights on for 30 minutes after wrapping them in a plastic wrap.

3. To prepare the filling, in a non-stick pan, put very little salt water, boil the spinach or simply sauté them on low heat or cook them in the steam. Squeeze and chop them finely. The spinach will weigh 100 gr once cooked and well squeezed.

4. In a bowl, put the chopped spinach in which you will add the parmesan and ricotta, salt, pepper and nutmeg. Use a soft but compact mixture to mix all the ingredients.

5. In a very thin sheet, roll out the egg pasta which you will cut into rectangles measuring 10x8 cm. Put a little teaspoon of filling in every rectangle of pasta and on a longer side, wrap the dough on itself.

6. Model your sweets by turning the left flap counterclockwise and the right flap clockwise as though to close the paper of the candy. Using a serrated wheel cut the outer edges of both edges.

7. After modeling all the candies, put them to dry on a floured work surface for an hour. In salted boiling water, cook the pasta for at least 5 minutes.

8. Let the sage leaves gild in melted butter in a pan.

9. Drain the candies once cooked and season them with sage and butter and grated parmesan to taste.

10. Your spinach and ricotta candies are ready to be served.

Nutrition: Calories: 458 Sugar: 2 g Fat: 23 g Carbohydrates: 1 g Fiber: 13 g Protein: 78 g.

19.Broccoli Pasta With Lemon And Kale

Preparation time: 10 minutes

Cooking time: 10 minutes

Serves: 4

Ingredients:

- 2 tablespoons extra-virgin olive oil
- 1/2 medium yellow onion, diced
- 1 garlic clove, minced
- 1 head broccoli, cut into florets, stem spiralized
- Salt
- Freshly ground black pepper
- 3 to 4 cups curly kale, chopped
- Juice of 2 lemons
- 1/4 teaspoon crushed red pepper

Directions:

1. In a large skillet over medium heat, heat the olive oil and sauté the onion and garlic for about 5 minutes, until translucent. Add the broccoli florets and spiralized stems and stir to combine. Season with salt and pepper.

2. Add the kale to the pan and stir until it begins to wilt, about 3 minutes. Add the lemon juice, crushed red pepper, and a bit more salt and pepper if necessary. Cook for 3 to 4 minutes more, or until the kale is wilted and tender. Serve immediately.

Nutrition: Calories 123 Fat 7g, Protein 4g, Sodium 342mg, Carbs 1.2g, Fiber 3g

20. Broccoli Ramen Bowl

Preparation time: 15 minutes

Cooking time: 2 hours

Serves: 4

Ingredients:

- 1 pound pork tenderloin
- 1 tablespoon salt
- 2 bunches green onions, (11/2 chopped for the broth, 1/2 sliced for garnish)
- 1 (2-inch) piece peeled fresh ginger, sliced (about 2 tablespoons)
- 4 garlic cloves, crushed
- 7 cups water
- 3 eggs, for topping
- Jalapeño peppers, for topping
- Bean sprouts, for topping
- Fresh cilantro, for topping
- 5 tablespoons coconut aminos
- 2 tablespoons rice vinegar
- 11/2 tablespoons sesame oil
- 2 or 3 broccoli stems, spiralized (reserve florets for another recipe)

Directions:

1. Season the pork with a generous sprinkling of salt and refrigerate overnight.

2. Place the pork in a large saucepan. Add the 11/2 bunches green onions to the pot with the ginger, garlic, and water. Bring to a boil, turn the heat down to a simmer, and cook for at least 2 hours (or up to 4 hours).

3. While the broth is simmering, prepare your toppings. Hard-boil the eggs (place in a pot of boiling water and cook for 10 minutes; cool under running water, peel, and halve), slice the jalapeños, and chop the bean sprouts and cilantro.

4. Add the coconut aminos, rice vinegar, and sesame oil to the broth. Continue to simmer and add the broccoli noodles about 5 minutes before you're ready to serve.

5. Remove the pork, slice it, and then transfer it back to the saucepan. Serve the ramen topped with 1/2 hard-boiled egg per bowl, sliced jalapeño, and chopped bean sprouts and cilantro.

Nutrition: Calories 171 Fat 6g, Protein 22g, Sodium 1,230mg, Carbs 5g, Fiber 2g

21.BEEF And BROCCOLI NOODLES

Preparation time: 10 minutes

Cooking time: 20 minutes

Serves: 4

Ingredients:

- 1 tablespoon grass-fed butter
- 1/2 medium yellow onion, diced
- 2 garlic cloves, minced
- 1 tablespoon sesame oil
- 1 pound steak, sliced thin
- 1 head broccoli, cut into florets, stem spiralized
- 2 tablespoons coconut aminos
- 1/4 teaspoon crushed red pepper
- 2 tablespoons sesame seeds, for garnish
- 2 or 3 green onions, finely chopped, for garnish

Directions:

1. In a large skillet or wok over medium heat, melt the butter. Add the onion and garlic and sauté for about 5 minutes, until translucent, before adding the sesame oil and steak. Cook for another 5 to 6 minutes, or until the meat begins to brown on all sides.

2. Chop the broccoli florets into bite-size pieces and add them to the skillet. Cook for 3 to 4 minutes and then add the broccoli noodles. Stir to combine and add the coconut aminos and crushed red pepper.

3. Remove from the heat and serve garnished with sesame seeds and green onions.

Nutrition: Calories 347 Fat 15g, Protein 45g, Sodium 397mg, Carbs 5g, Fiber 3g

22.   Beef Stroganoff

Preparation time: 10 minutes

Cooking time: 30 minutes

Serves: 6

Ingredients:

- 4 tablespoons grass-fed butter, divided
- 1 large yellow onion, sliced thin
- 2 garlic cloves, minced
- 11/2 pounds beef sirloin steak, sliced
- Salt
- Freshly ground black pepper
- 1 cup beef broth
- 1/2 cup canned coconut milk
- 2 large broccoli stems, spiralized

Directions:

1. In a large skillet over medium heat, melt 1 tablespoon of butter. Sauté the onion and garlic for about 5 minutes, until translucent. Add another tablespoon of butter and the steak. Cook until the meat is browned on all sides, about 5 minutes. Season with salt and pepper.

2. Add the broth and coconut milk to the skillet and stir well to combine. Bring to a simmer and cook on low for about 10 minutes, or until the liquid has thickened a bit.

3. While the beef is simmering, bring a small saucepan of water to a boil. Add the broccoli noodles and cook for 2 to 3

minutes, or until tender. Drain and toss with the remaining 2 tablespoons of butter.

4. Transfer the noodles to plates, top with the beef and sauce, and serve.

Nutrition: Calories 525 Fat 30g, Protein 55g, Sodium 696mg, Carbs 3g, Fiber 3g

KETO CHAFFLE

23. Chicken Jalapeno Chaffle

Servings: 4

PreparationTime:5minutes

Cooking time 8–10 minutes

Ingredients

- Batter
- ½ pound ground chicken
- 4 eggs
- cup grated mozzarella cheese
- tablespoons sour cream
- green jalapeno, chopped
- Salt and pepper to taste
- teaspoon dried oregano
- ½ teaspoon dried garlic
- Other
- tablespoons butter to brush the waffle maker
- ¼ cup sour cream to garnish
- 1 green jalapeno, diced, to garnish

Directions

1. Preheat the waffle maker.

2. Add the ground chicken, eggs, mozzarella cheese, sour cream, chopped jalapeno, salt and pepper, dried oregano and dried garlic to a bowl.

3. Mix everything until batter forms.

4. Brush the heated waffle maker with butter and add a few tablespoons of the batter.

5. Close the lid and cook for about 8–10 minutes depending on your waffle maker.

6. Serve with a tablespoon of sour cream and sliced jalapeno on top.

Nutrition (per serving) Calories 284, fat 19.4 g, carbs 2.2 g, sugar 0.6 g, Protein 24.7 g, sodium 204 mg

24. Turkey BBQ Sauce Chaffle

Servings: 4

PreparationTime:5minutes

Cooking time 8–10 minutes

Ingredients

- Batter
- ½ pound ground turkey meat
- 3 eggs
- cup grated Swiss cheese
- ¼ cup cream cheese
- ¼ cup BBQ sauce
- teaspoon dried oregano
- Salt and pepper to taste
- cloves garlic, minced
- Other
- tablespoons butter to brush the waffle maker
- ¼ cup BBQ sauce for serving
- tablespoons freshly chopped parsley for garnish

Directions

1. Preheat the waffle maker.
2. Add the ground turkey, eggs, grated Swiss cheese, cream cheese, BBQ sauce, dried oregano, salt and pepper, and minced garlic to a bowl.
3. Mix everything until combined and batter forms.

4. Brush the heated waffle maker with butter and add a few tablespoons of the batter.

5. Close the lid and cook for about 8–10 minutes depending on your waffle maker.

6. Serve each chaffle with a tablespoon of BBQ sauce and a sprinkle of freshly chopped parsley.

Nutrition (per serving) Calories 365, fat 23.7 g, carbs 13.7 g, sugar 8.8 g, Protein 23.5 g, sodium 595 mg

25. Classic Beef Chaffle

Servings: 4

PreparationTime:5minutes

Cooking time 10 minutes

Ingredients

- Batter
- ½ pound ground beef
- 4 eggs
- 4 ounces cream cheese
- cup grated mozzarella cheese
- Salt and pepper to taste
- clove garlic, minced
- ½ teaspoon freshly chopped rosemary
- Other
- tablespoons butter to brush the waffle maker
- ¼ cup sour cream
- tablespoons freshly chopped parsley for garnish

Directions

a. Preheat the waffle maker.

b. Add the ground beef, eggs, cream cheese, grated mozzarella cheese, salt and pepper, minced garlic and freshly chopped rosemary to a bowl.

c. Brush the heated waffle maker with butter and add a few tablespoons of the batter.

d. Close the lid and cook for about 8–10 minutes depending on your waffle maker.

e. Serve each chaffle with a tablespoon of sour cream and freshly chopped parsley on top.

f. Serve and enjoy.

Nutrition (per serving) Calories 368, fat 27.4 g, carbs 2.1 g, sugar 0.4 g, Protein 27.4 g, sodium 291 mg

26.   Beef and Sour Cream Chaffle

Servings: 4

PreparationTime:5minutes

Cooking time 15 minutes

Ingredients

- Batter
- 4 eggs
- 2 cups grated mozzarella cheese
- 3 tablespoons coconut flour
- 3 tablespoons almond flour
- 2 teaspoons baking powder
- Salt and pepper to taste
- tablespoon freshly chopped parsley
- Seasoned beef
- pound beef tenderloin
- Salt and pepper to taste
- tablespoons olive oil
- tablespoon Dijon mustard
- Other
- tablespoons olive oil to brush the waffle maker
- ¼ cup sour cream for garnish
- tablespoons freshly chopped spring onion for garnish

Directions

1. Preheat the waffle maker.

2. Add the eggs, grated mozzarella cheese, coconut flour, almond flour, baking powder, salt and pepper and freshly chopped parsley to a bowl.

3. Mix until just combined and batter forms.

4. Brush the heated waffle maker with olive oil and add a few tablespoons of the batter.

5. Close the lid and cook for about 5–7 minutes depending on your waffle maker.

6. Meanwhile, heat the olive oil in a nonstick pan over medium heat.

7. Season the beef tenderloin with salt and pepper and spread the whole piece of beef tenderloin with Dijon mustard.

8. Cook on each side for about 4–5 minutes.

9. Serve each chaffle with sour cream and slices of the cooked beef tenderloin.

10. Garnish with freshly chopped spring onion.

11. Serve and enjoy.

Nutrition (per serving) Calories 543, fat 37 g, carbs 7.9 g, sugar 0.5 g, Protein 44.9 g, sodium 269 mg

27.   Beef and Tomato Chaffle

Servings: 4

PreparationTime:5minutes

Cooking time 15 minutes

Ingredients

- Batter
- 4 eggs
- ¼ cup cream cheese
- cup grated mozzarella cheese
- Salt and pepper to taste
- ¼ cup almond flour
- teaspoon freshly chopped dill
- Beef
- pound beef loin
- Salt and pepper to taste
- 1 tablespoon balsamic vinegar
- tablespoons olive oil
- 1 teaspoon freshly chopped rosemary
- Other
- tablespoons cooking spray to brush the waffle maker
- tomato slices for serving

Directions

1. Preheat the waffle maker.

2. Add the eggs, cream cheese, grated mozzarella cheese, salt and pepper, almond flour and freshly chopped dill to a bowl.

3. Mix until combined and batter forms.

4. Brush the heated waffle maker with cooking spray and add a few tablespoons of the batter.

5. Close the lid and cook for about 8–10 minutes depending on your waffle maker.

6. Meanwhile, heat the olive oil in a nonstick frying pan and season the beef loin with salt and pepper and freshly chopped rosemary.

7. Cook the beef on each side for about 5 minutes and drizzle with some balsamic vinegar.

8. Serve each chaffle with a slice of tomato and cooked beef loin slices.

Nutrition (per serving) Calories 492, fat 35.8 g, carbs 3.3 g, sugar 0.8 g, Protein 40.3 g, sodium 200 mg

28.   Beef Chaffle Sandwich Recipe

Servings: 4

PreparationTime:5minutes

Cooking time 15 minutes

Ingredients

- Batter
- 3 eggs
- 2 cups grated mozzarella cheese
- ¼ cup cream cheese
- Salt and pepper to taste
- teaspoon Italian seasoning
- Beef
- tablespoons butter
- pound beef tenderloin
- Salt and pepper to taste
- teaspoons Dijon mustard
- teaspoon dried paprika
- Other
- tablespoons cooking spray to brush the waffle maker
- lettuce leaves for serving
- tomato slices for serving
- leaves fresh basil

Directions

1.   Preheat the waffle maker.

2.   Add the eggs, grated mozzarella cheese, salt and pepper and Italian seasoning to a bowl.

3.   Mix until combined and batter forms.

4.   Brush the heated waffle maker with cooking spray and add a few tablespoons of the batter.

5.   Close the lid and cook for about 5–7 minutes depending on your waffle maker.

6.   Meanwhile, melt and heat the butter in a nonstick frying pan.

7.   Season the beef loin with salt and pepper, brush it with Dijon mustard, and sprinkle some dried paprika on top.

8.   Cook the beef on each side for about 5 minutes.

9.   Thinly slice the beef and assemble the chaffle sandwiches.

10.   Cut each chaffle in half and on one half place a lettuce leaf, tomato slice, basil leaf, and some sliced beef.

11.   Cover with the other chaffle half and serve.

Nutrition (per serving) Calories 477, fat 32.8g, carbs 2.3 g, sugar 0.9 g, Protein 42.2 g, sodium 299 mg

KETO BREAD MACHINE

29. Cinnamon Flavored Bread

Preparation Time: 35-40 minutes

Cooking Time: 0 minutes

Servings: 8 slices

Ingredients:

- 1 lb. almond flour
- 1 oz. coconut flour
- 2 oz. flaxseeds (ground)
- 5 eggs
- 1/2 tbsp. vinegar (apple cider)
- 1/8 tbsp. salt
- 1/3 tbsp. of baking soda
- 2 tbsp. honey
- 3 tbsp. butter
- 3 tsp. cinnamon
- 1/2 tsp. chia seeds

Directions:

1. Heat the oven beforehand to a temperature of 350 degrees Fahrenheit. Lay a piece of parchment paper on the bottom part of an eight-by-four bread pan and oil the sides of the pan.

2. Take a large bowl and mix coconut flour, almond flour, baking soda, ground flaxseeds, salt, and one and a half teaspoon cinnamon in it.

3. Whisk the eggs in another bowl. Then add honey, vinegar, and two tablespoons butter in it.

4. Mix the wet items into the dry ones and prepare the batter. Make sure that there are no bulges in the coconut or almond flours.

5. Dispense the batter into the greased pan and bake for 30 to 35 minutes. Take it out of the oven.

6. Whisk one tablespoon of butter and mix one and a half teaspoon of cinnamon in it. Brush this mixture on the bread.

7. Allow it to cool and then serve.

Nutrition: Calories: 221 Total fats: 15.4 grams Carbohydrates: 1.7 grams Fiber: 3.1 grams Sugar: 3.7 grams Protein: 9.3 grams

MAINS

30. Healthy Halibut Fillets

Preparation Time: 5 minutes

Cooking Time: 10 minutes

Servings: 2

Ingredients:

- 2 Halibut fillets
- tbsp Dill
- tbsp Onion powder
- cup Parsley, chopped
- tbsp Paprika
- 1 tbsp Garlic powder
- 1 tbsp Lemon Pepper
- tbsp Lemon juice

Directions:

1. Mix lemon juice, lemon pepper, garlic powder, and paprika, parsley, dill and onion powder in a bowl. Pour the mixture in the Instant pot and place the halibut fish over it.
2. Seal the lid, press Manual mode and cook for 10 minutes on High pressure. When ready, do a quick pressure release by setting the valve to venting.

Nutrition: Calories 283, Protein 22.5g, Net Carbs 6.2g, Fat 16.4g

31.Clean Salmon with Soy Sauce

Preparation Time: 10 minutes

Cooking Time: 30 minutes

Servings: 2

Ingredients:

- 2 Salmon fillets
- 2 tbsp Avocado oil
- 2 tbsp Soy sauce
- tbsp Garlic powder
- tbsp fresh Dill to garnish
- Salt and Pepper, to taste

Directions:

1. To make the marinade, thoroughly mix the soy sauce, avocado oil, salt, pepper and garlic powder into a bowl. Dip salmon in the mixture and place in the refrigerator for 20 minutes.

2. Transfer the contents to the Instant pot. Seal, set on Manual and cook for 10 minutes on high pressure. When ready, do a quick release. Serve topped with the fresh dill.

Nutrition: Calories 512, Protein 65g, Net Carbs 3.2g, Fat 21g

32. Faux Beet Risotto

Preparation Time: 5 minutes

Cooking Time: 15 minutes

Servings: 2

Ingredients:

- 4 Beets, tails and leafs removed
- 2 tbsp Olive oil
- big head Cauliflower, cut into florets
- 4 tbsp cup Full Milk
- tsp Red Chili Flakes
- Salt to taste
- Black Pepper to taste
- ½ cup Water

Directions:

1. Pour the water in the Instant Pot and fit a steamer basket. Place the beets and cauliflower in the basket. Seal the lid, and cook on High Pressure mode for 4 minutes.

2. Once ready, do a natural pressure release for 10 minutes, then quickly release the pressure.Remove the steamer basket with the vegetables and discard water. Remove the beets' peels.

3. Place veggies back to the pot, add salt, pepper, and flakes. Mash with a potato masher. Hit Sauté, and cook the milk for 2 minutes. Stir frequently. Dish onto plates and drizzle with oil.

Nutrition: Calories 153, Protein 3.6g, Net Carbs 2.5g, Fat 9g

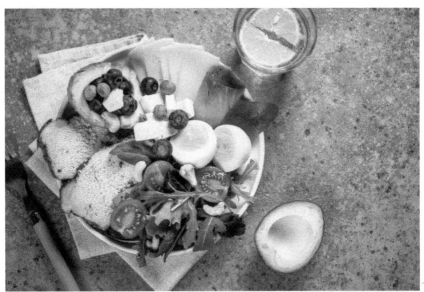

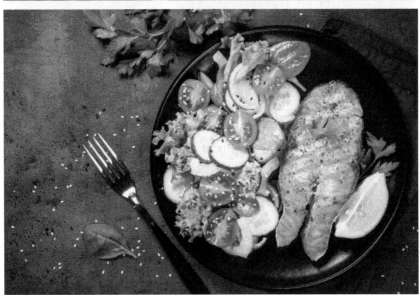

SIDES

33. Lemon Parsnips Mix

Preparation Time: 10 minutes

Cooking Time: 35 minutes

Servings: 6

Ingredients:

- 2 pound parsnips, cut into medium chunks
- 2 tablespoons lemon peel, grated
- cup veggie stock
- A pinch of salt and black pepper
- tablespoons olive oil
- ¼ cup cilantro, chopped

Directions:

1. Heat up a pan with the oil at medium-high heat, add the parsnips, stir and brown them for 5 minutes.
2. Add lemon peel, stock, salt, pepper and cilantro, stir, cover the pan, reduce heat to medium and cook for 30 minutes.
3. Divide the mix between then serve.

Nutrition: Calories: 179 kcal Fat: 4 Fiber: 4 Carbs: 6 Protein; 8

34.   Mustard Cabbage

Preparation Time: 10 minutes

Cooking Time: 20 minutes

Servings: 4

Ingredients:

- onion, sliced
- cabbage head, shredded
- A pinch of salt and black pepper
- cup chicken stock
- tablespoons mustard
- 1 tablespoon olive oil

Directions:

1. Heat up a pan with the oil at medium-high heat, add the onion, stir and cook for 5 minutes.

2. Add the cabbage, salt, pepper, stock and mustard, stir, cook for 15 minutes, divide between plates and serve as a side dish.

Nutrition: Calories: 197 Fat: 4 Fiber: 2 Carbs: 8 Protein: 5

VEGETABLES

35.   Garlic Brussels sprouts with Bacon

Preparation time: 5 minutes

Cooking time: 15 minutes

Servings: 2

Ingredients:

- 3 slices of bacon

- 4 oz Brussels sprouts, halved

- 2 green onions, diced

- ¾ tbsp butter, unsalted

- 2 tbsp chicken broth

- ½ tsp garlic powder

- ¼ tsp salt

- ¾ tbsp avocado oil

Directions:

1.   Take a medium skillet pan, place it over medium heat, add oil and wait until it gets hot.

2.   Cut bacon slices into squares, add to the skillet pan and cook for 2 to 3 minutes until bacon fat starts to render.

3.   Transfer bacon pieces to a plate lined with paper towels and then set aside until required.

4. Add butter into the skillet pan and when it starts to brown, add onion, sprinkle with garlic powder and cook for 1 minute or more until semi-translucent.

5. Add sprouts, season with salt, stir until mixed and cook for 2 to 3 minutes until beginning to brown.

6. Pour in chicken broth, stir until mixed and cook for 5 to 7 minutes until broth is absorbed, covering the pan.

7. Then make a hole in the center of pan by pushing sprouts to the side of the pan, add bacon and stir until well mixed.

8. Serve.

Nutrition: 202 Calories; 15.1 g Fats; 7.7 g Protein; 3.9 g Net Carb; 2.4 g Fiber;

36.   Spanish-Style "Tortilla de Patatas"

Preparation Time: 10 minutes

Cooking Time: 20 minutes

Servings: 3

Ingredients:

- 5 eggs, beaten

- cup spinach, torn, rinsed

- potato, chopped

- cup heavy cream

- Salt and black pepper to taste

- ¼ tsp dried thyme

- 1 tbsp. olive oil

Directions:

1. In a bowl, mix eggs, heavy cream, and potato. Dust with salt and black pepper, and stir to combine. Heat oil on Sauté and cook the spinach and thyme for 3 minutes, or until wilted. Remove the spinach from the pot.

2. Stir in the spinach in the previously prepared mixture. Transfer all to an oven-safe dish that fits in the instant pot. Add 1 cup of water, insert the trivet, pour 1 cup of water, and place the oven-safe dish on top. Close the lid then cook on High Pressure for at least 20 minutes. Release the steam naturally, for 5 minutes.

Nutrition: Calories: 524 kcal Protein: 20.97 g Fat: 37.57 g Carbohydrates: 26.09 g

37.   English Vegetable Potage

Preparation Time: 10 minutes

Cooking Time: 45 minutes

Servings: 4

Ingredients:

- lb. potatoes, peeled, cut into bite-sized pieces
- carrots, peeled, chopped
- celery stalks, chopped
- 2 onions, peeled, chopped
- zucchini, chopped into ½ -inch thick slices
- A handful of fresh celery leaves
- tbsp. butter, unsalted
- tbsp. olive oil
- 2 cups vegetable broth
- tbsp. paprika
- Salt and black pepper to taste
- bay leaves

Directions:

1. Warm oil on Sauté and stir-fry the onions for 3-4 minutes, until translucent. Add carrots, celery, zucchini, and ¼ cup of broth. Continue to cook for at least 10 minutes more, stirring constantly.

2. Stir in potatoes, paprika, salt, pepper, bay leaves, remaining broth, and celery leaves. Seal the lid and cook on Meat/Stew

mode for 30 minutes on High. Do a quick release and stir in butter.

Nutrition: Calories: 1260 kcal Protein: 6 g Fat: 126.94 g Carbohydrates: 36.56 g

38. Keto white pizza with mushrooms and pesto

Preparation Time: 10 minutes

Cooking Time: 20 minutes

Servings: 2

Ingredients:

- For the crust
- 2 eggs
- 3/4 cup almond flour
- teaspoon baking powder
- tablespoon psyllium husk powder
- 1/2 cup mayonnaise
- 1/2 teaspoon salt
- For the topping
- ounces mushrooms (finely sliced)
- 1/2 cup sour cream
- tablespoon green pesto
- 3/4 cup shredded cheese
- tablespoon olive oil
- Salt and pepper, to taste

Directions:

1. Preheat the oven to 350 degrees Fahrenheit
2. Beat the eggs in a large bowl and add mayonnaise to it.
3. Whisk together until you get a frothy and creamy mixture

4. Add the almond flour, baking powder, psyllium husk powder, and salt to the egg-mayonnaise mixture

5. Mix thoroughly until the contents are blended well and let it sit for 5 minutes.

6. Line a baking tray with parchment and then move the crust mixture into it.

7. Using a spatula spread out the mixture equally to prepare the crust (should be around 1/2 inch thick)

8. Bake for 10 minutes until the crust turns light golden brown – don't overdo and burn it.

9. Take off the crust from the oven then let it cool for 10 minutes.

10. Once cooled, turn out the crust into a cutting board and slowly remove the parchment paper

11. Place the sliced mushrooms into a small bowl and add the pesto into it.

12. Mix them well as you slowly add the olive oil too. Season with pepper and salt.

13. Combine the contents thoroughly until the flavors blend well

14. Layer out the sour cream on the prepared crust and top it with the shredded cheese

15. Now add the mushroom mixture and spread it out evenly

16. Use the same parchment paper to line the baking tray and place the pizza onto it

17. Return the pizza to the oven and let it back for 10 minutes until the cheese melts.

18. Turn off the heat and slice out the pizza. Transfer to a plate and serve warm. Enjoy!

Nutrition: Calories 1147 Kcal Fat: 110 g Protein: 27 g Net carb: 7 g

SOUPS AND STEWS

39. Roasted Poblano and Cheddar Soup

Preparation Time: 11 minutes

Cooking Time: 15 minutes

Servings: 4

Ingredients:

- 2 medium poblano peppers
- ½ medium cauliflower, broken into pieces
    - o   cups vegetable stock
- tbsp. butter
- ¼ cup diced onion
- ¼-cup sour cream
- cup + 2 tbsp. shredded cheddar cheese
- tbsp. garlic powder
- 1 tsp cumin & 1 tsp smoked paprika

Directions:

1. Set the broiler to high and put the poblano peppers on a baking sheet.

2. Roast the poblano pepper, occasionally turning for even cooking until the skins are dark and the peppers are tender.

3. Place peppers in a jar with a lid and seal to cool. Set aside, meanwhile prepare the soup base.

4. On the stovetop or in the microwave, steam cauliflower florets until very tender for about 5 minutes or 7-10 on the stovetop.

5. In a high-speed blender or food processor, blend steamed cauliflower and 1 cup stock. Pour in the remaining stock and continue to process until the mixture is smooth and creamy.

6. In a shallow pot, heat the butter and onion until translucent.

7. Pour in half the cauliflower puree, cheese, and sour cream to the pot and stir until thickened. Reduce to low heat.

8. Dice the peel and deseeded poblano pepper, reserving about 1 tbsp. add the pepper into the soup. Pour in the remaining cauliflower mixture and simmer for about 4-6 minutes.

9. Stir in the smoked paprika, garlic powder, and cumin and remove from heat.

Nutrition: 241 Calories 16 g Fat 10 g Carbohydrates 10 g Protein

40. Cabbage Creamy Soup

Preparation Time: 5 minutes

Cooking Time: 25 minutes

Servings: 5

Ingredients:

- 4 cups chopped cabbage
- 4 cups chicken stock
- cup heavy cream
- 4 slices bacon, cooked and crumbled

Directions:

1. Bring the chicken stock to boil over medium-high heat.
2. Add the cabbage.
3. Reduce the heat to low and simmer for 20-25 minutes or until the cabbage is tender. Stir in the heavy cream and simmer for 5 minutes. Serve hot, topped with crumbled bacon.

Nutrition: Calories 156 Fat 14.3 g Carbs 3.7 g Protein 4.1 g

41.Chicken Tomato Sausage Stew

Preparation Time: 10 minutes

Cooking Time: 30 minutes

Servings: 2-4

Ingredients:

- tablespoon coconut oil
- 1-pound Andouille pork sausage
- medium white onion, thinly sliced
- 6 cups tomatoes, chopped
- 4-pound chicken thighs, boneless, skinless
- bell peppers, diced
- celery stalks, chopped
- cups water or bone broth
- large carrots, chopped
- 6 garlic cloves, minced
- /4 cup parsley, minced
- teaspoon thyme
- 1 teaspoon salt
- 1/2 teaspoon red chili flakes, crushed
- 1/2 teaspoon smoked paprika
- 1/4 teaspoon cayenne
- 1/4 teaspoon black pepper hot sauce (if desired
- 1 bay leaf

Directions:

1. Put coconut oil into Instant Pot. Press "Sauté" button, put sausage and chicken into Instant Pot and sauté till the meat is evenly cooked. Take out cooked meat and set aside.

2. Put celery, onions, bell peppers, and carrots into Instant Pot.

3. Press "Sauté" button and stir from time to time.

4. Put minced garlic into Instant Pot and continue sautéing.

5. Put chopped tomatoes and broth into Instant Pot.

6. Continue sautéing until simmering.

7. Once cooled, slice sausage and chicken into small chunks.

8. Put sausage, chicken, spices and the minced parsley into Instant Pot, stir until evenly mixed.

9. Close the lid, and turn the vent to "Sealed".

10. Press "Soup" button, set the timer for 5-10 minutes and set "Pressure" to high.

11. Once the timer is up press "Cancel" button and turn the steam release handle to "Venting" position for quick release, until the float valve drops down.

12. Open the lid.

13. Serve warm, topped with hot sauce (if desired).

Nutrition: Calories: 1414 kcal Protein: 93.65 g Fat: 103.44 g Carbohydrates: 25.49 g

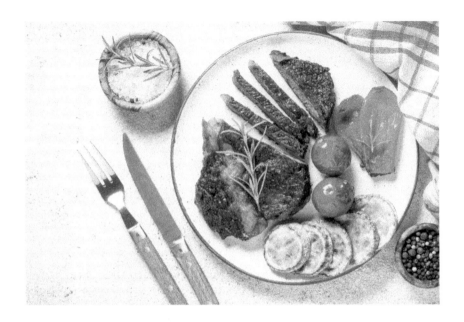

DRESSING AND SAUCES

42. Enchilada Sauce

Preparation Time: 10 minutes

Cooking Time: 10 minutes

Servings: 6

Ingredients:

- 3 ounces salted butter
- 1½ tablespoons Erythritol
- 2 teaspoons dried oregano
- 3 teaspoons ground cumin
- 2 teaspoons ground coriander
- 2 teaspoons onion powder
- ¼ teaspoon cayenne pepper
- Salt and ground black pepper, as required
- 12 ounces tomato puree

Directions:

1. Melt the butter in a medium pan over medium heat and sauté all the ingredients except tomato puree for about 3 minutes.

2. Add the tomato puree and simmer for about 5 minutes.

3. Remove the pan from heat and let it cool slightly before serving.

4. You can preserve this sauce in the refrigerator by placing it into an airtight container.

Nutrition: Calories: 132 Net Carbs: 5.1g Carbohydrate: 6.6g Fiber: 1.5g Protein: 1.4g Fat: 11.9g Sugar: 3.1g Sodium: 127mg

DESSERT

43. Spicy Almond Fat Bombs

Preparation time: 10 minutes

Cooking time: 4 minutes

Servings: 3

Ingredients:

- ¾ cup coconut oil
- ¼ cup almond butter
- ¼ cup cocoa powder
- 3 drops liquid stevia
- ⅛ teaspoon chili powder
- Special equipment:
- A 12-cup muffin pan

Directions:

1. Line a muffin pan with 12 paper liners. Keep aside.
2. Heat the oil in a small saucepan over low heat, then add the almond butter, cocoa powder, stevia, and chili powder. Stir to combine well.
3. Divide the mixture evenly among the muffin cups and keep the muffin pan in the refrigerator for 15 minutes, or until the bombs are set and firm.

4. Serve immediately or refrigerate to chill until ready to serve.

Nutrition: calories: 160 fat: 16.8g total carbs: 2.0g fiber: 1.2g protein: 1.5g

44.   Chocolate Granola Bars

Preparation time: 10 minutes

Cooking time: 20 minutes

Servings: 20

Ingredients:

- 3 ounces (85 g) almonds
- 3 ounces (85 g) walnuts
- 2 ounces (57 g) sesame seeds
- 2 ounces (57 g) pumpkin seeds
- ounce (28 g) flaxseed
- ounces (57 g) unsweetened coconut, shredded
- ounces (57 g) dark chocolate with a minimum of 70% cocoa solids
- 6 tablespoons coconut oil
- tablespoons tahini
- teaspoon vanilla extract
- teaspoons ground cinnamon
- pinch sea salt
- eggs

Directions:

1. Preheat your oven to 350°F (180°C).
2. Except for dark chocolate, process all the ingredients for granola in a food processor until they make a coarse and crumbly mixture.

3. Spread the granola mixture into a greased baking dish lined with parchment paper.

4. Bake the granola for 15 to 20 minutes in the oven until the cake turns golden brown.

5. Once baked, allow it to cool for 5 minutes, then remove from the baking dish.

6. Cut the granola cake into 24 bars using a sharp knife on a clean work surface. Set aside.

7. Melt the chocolate by heating in a double boiler or in the microwave. Let it cool for 5 minutes.

8. Serve the granola bars with the melted chocolate for dipping.

Nutrition: calories: fat: 17.2g total carbs: 7.0g fiber: 3.2g protein: 4.7g

45.   Keto Lava Cake

Preparation time: 15 minutes

Cooking time: 10 minutes

Servings: 6

Ingredients:

- tablespoon melted butter, for greasing the ramekins
- ounces (57 g) dark chocolate with a minimum of 70% cocoa solids
- ounces (57 g) butter
- ¼ teaspoon vanilla extract
- eggs
- Special equipment:
- to 6 small ramekins

Directions:

1. Preheat your oven to 400°F (205°C) and lightly grease 4 to 6 small ramekins with 1 tablespoon melted butter.

2. Cut the chocolate into small pieces on your cutting board. Add the chocolate and butter to a double broiler, and heat until they are melted. Mix well.

3. Add the vanilla to the chocolate mixture, then allow the mixture to cool.

4. Beat all the eggs in a mixing bowl for 3 minutes until fluffy, then add the chocolate mixture. Stir to combine.

5. Divide the mixture among the greased ramekins. Bake all the ramekins in the preheated oven for 5 minutes.

6. Remove from the oven and cool for 5 minutes before enjoying.

Nutrition: calories: 197 fat: 17.8g total carbs: 4.9g fiber: 1.0g protein: 5.4g

46.   Coco Avocado Truffles

Preparation time: 35 minutes

Cooking time:

Servings: 20

Ingredients:

- ripe avocado, chopped

- ½ teaspoon vanilla extract

- ½ lime zest

- pinch salt

- 5 ounces (142 g) dark chocolate with a minimum of 80% cocoa solids, finely chopped

- tablespoon coconut oil

- 1 tablespoon unsweetened cocoa powder

Directions:

1. In a bowl, thoroughly mix the avocado flesh with vanilla extract with an electric hand mixer until it forms a smooth mixture.

2. Add the lime zest and a pinch of salt, then mix well. Set aside.

3. Mix and melt the chocolate with coconut oil in a double broiler or by heating in the microwave.

4. Add the chocolate mixture to the avocado mash. Blend well until a smooth batter forms.

5. Refrigerate this batter for 30 minutes until firm.

6. Scoop portions of the batter (about 2 teaspoons in size) and shape into small truffle balls with your hands, then roll each truffle ball in the cocoa powder. Serve immediately.

Nutrition: calories: 61 fat: 5.2g total carbs: 4.3g fiber: 1.6g protein: 0.8g

47. Pumpkin Spice Fat Bombs

Preparation Time: 10 minutes + 1 hour freezing

Cooking Time: 0 minutes

Servings: 16

Ingredients:

- ½ cup butter, at room temperature
- ½ cup cream cheese, at room temperature
- ⅓ cup pure pumpkin purée
- 3 tablespoons chopped almonds
- 4 drops liquid stevia
- ½ teaspoon ground cinnamon
- ¼ teaspoon ground nutmeg

Directions:

1. Line an 8-by-8-inch pan with parchment paper and set aside.
2. In a small bowl, whisk together the butter and cream cheese until very smooth.
3. Add the pumpkin purée and whisk until blended.
4. Stir in the almonds, stevia, cinnamon, and nutmeg.
5. Spoon the pumpkin mixture into the pan.
6. Use a spatula to spread it equally in the pan, then place it in the freezer for about 1 hour.
7. Cut into 16 pieces and store the fat bombs in a tightly sealed container in the freezer until ready to serve.

Nutrition: Calories: 87 Fat,: 9g Protein: 1g Carbs: 1g Fiber: 0g Net Carbs: 1g

48. Creamy Banana Fat Bombs

Preparation Time: 10 minutes + 1 hour chilling

Cooking Time: 0 minutes

Servings: 4

Ingredients:

- 1¼ cups cream cheese, at room temperature
- ¾ cup heavy (whipping) cream
- tablespoon pure banana extract
- 6 drops liquid stevia

Directions:

1. Line a baking sheet using parchment paper then set aside.

2. In a medium bowl, beat together the cream cheese, heavy cream, banana extract, and stevia until smooth and very thick, about 5 minutes.

3. Gently spoon the mixture onto the baking sheet in mounds, leaving some space between each mound, and place the baking sheet in the refrigerator until firm, about 1 hour.

Nutrition: Calories: 134 Fat,: 12g Protein: 3g Carbs: 1g Fiber: 0g Net Carbs: 1g

49.   <u>Lemon-Lime Bars</u>

Preparation Time: 20 minutes + chilling time

Cooking Time: 35 minutes

Servings: 4

Ingredients:

- Crust

- ¾ cup almond flour

- ½ cup butter

- ½ cup erythritol-stevia blend

- ¼ cup coconut flour

- ½ teaspoon sea salt

- Filling

- 3 eggs

- 2 tablespoons fresh lemon juice

- 2 tablespoons fresh lime juice

- ½ cup erythritol-stevia blend

- ½ teaspoon baking powder

- ½ teaspoon pure vanilla extract

- ¼ teaspoon sea salt

- Topping

- Zest from lemon

- Zest from lime

Directions:

1. You make the crust first - preheat your oven to 325-degrees.

2. Prepare a glass pan with a coconut-oil based spray.

3. Mix all the crust ingredients together.

4. Press into the bottom of the pan and bake for 15 minutes.

5. Cool.

6. To make the filling, simply mix everything together.

7. When the crust is cool, pour overfilling.

8. Put back in the oven for 15 minutes.

9. Check to see if the bars look set.

10. If still liquidy and jiggly, bake for another 5 minutes.

11. Cool before chilling in the fridge for 25 minutes or so.

12. For an extra hit of citrus, sprinkle lemon and lime zest on top!

Nutrition: Total calories: 109 Protein: 3 Carbs: 3 Fat: 10 Fiber: 0

50. Macadamia Brownies

Preparation Time: 5 minutes + 30 minutes chilling

Cooking Time: 25 minutes

Servings: 12

Ingredients:

- 10 ½ tablespoons melted butter

- 8 tablespoons softened cream cheese

- 6 eggs

- 4 tablespoons unsweetened dark + natural (non-alkalized) cocoa powder

- 4 tablespoons Sukrin Gold

- 3 teaspoons pure vanilla extract

- ½ teaspoon baking powder

- Generous handful of crushed macadamia nuts

- Pinch of sea salt

Directions:

1. Preheat your oven to 350-degrees.

2. Put ingredients (minus walnuts) in a mixing bowl and blend together.

3. Fold in nuts.

4. Line a baking dish with parchment paper.

5. Pour in batter.

6. Bake for 20-25 minutes, until the brownies are solid and not liquidy at all.

7. Cool 30 minutes before cutting.

Nutrition: Total calories: 178 Protein: 4.5 Carbs: 3.5 Fat: 17 Fiber: 2

CONCLUSION

Keto can be a great option for people looking to shed extra weight that is stored in their bodies as fat. Ketosis is the process of the body using fats instead of glucose for energy. The liver can take fats and break them down into ketones, which can be used by both the body and the brain as a fuel source. To get the body away from using sugars, however, a person has to severely limit the amount and type of carbs they consume so the body can burn through its glucose stores and start working on the fat stores. This is why it can be so important to stay diligent on the diet once started; otherwise, a person might not see their desired results.

For people who are ready to dedicate themselves 100% to the keto diet, there are various forms of it that can match any person's lifestyle and goals. The standard keto option is best for people trying the diet for the first time because it can be the quickest way to get into ketosis and reap the immediate benefits. There are also cyclical and targeted keto for people who might not be willing to follow the strict diet every day. These options give people an opportunity to consume carbs on certain days based on their own personal plans.

There are many benefits to starting the keto diet beyond just losing weight. Keto can also help people improve their heart health by reducing bad fats and forcing the body to work through fats it has stored, possibly in dangerous places like arteries. It can also help people with certain types of epilepsy reduce seizures by switching the brain onto ketone power. Keto can also help women with PCOS regain their health by promoting weight loss and helping to balance their hormones, which can be a cause of the condition. It can even help clear up acne in some people by reducing blood sugar, which can improve skin conditions.

It is not difficult to switch to and stick to a Keto diet. What is actually difficult is adhering to strict rules and guidelines. As long as you maintain the Fats : Protein : Carbs ratio, you'll lose weight fast. It's a no-brainer. And quite unbecoming that many have deviated from this core principle of the Keto diet. The simple formula is to increase the fat and protein content in your meals and snacks while reducing your carb intake. You must restrict your carb intake to reach and remain in Ketosis. Different people achieve Ketosis with varying amounts of carb intake. Generally, it is easy to reach and stay in Ketosis when you decrease your carb intake to not more than 20grams.

Keeping keto long term can seem difficult for beginners who are just getting used to the mechanics of the diet, but it is not so difficult once they are acclimated to the keto lifestyle. Planning out meals and snacks can help people keep up keto longer because it takes some of the work and thinking out of dieting. A person can simply grab what they need and go. And if the standard keto doesn't work for someone long term, they can refer to the other keto styles to find one that will work for them beyond the initial diet.

CPSIA information can be obtained
at www.ICGtesting.com
Printed in the USA
BVHW040730100321
602119BV00006BA/1105